Take a Breath & Embrace Wellness

The COPD Companion

Essential Strategies for Managing Chronic Obstructive Pulmonary Disease Symptoms & Wellbeing

Jeffy E Flair

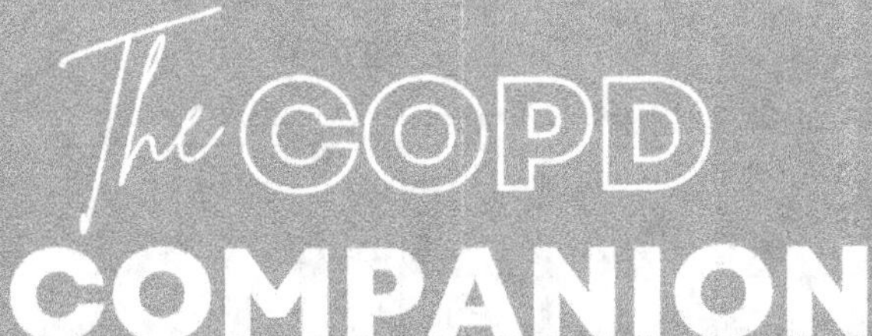

The COPD COMPANION

Essential Strategies for Managing Chronic Obstructive Pulmonary Disease Symptoms & Wellbeing

JEFFY E FLAIR

Content

INTRODUCTION

Imagine breathing as an ongoing uphill struggle rather than as a straightforward act. For millions of people suffering with Chronic Obstructive Pulmonary Disease (COPD), which is a complicated illness that affects not only the lungs but also every aspect of everyday life, this is their reality. COPD isn't a place we prefer to explore, in contrast to other landscapes.

It's a route that is forced upon us, frequently by avoidable means, yet it has unchangeable consequences. But do not be alarmed; there is more to this trip than just suffering. Let's take a thorough look at COPD, dispelling its myths and learning more about the significant impact it has on our lives. Together, we may negotiate this complex landscape in search of comprehension, empowerment, and a way to live well even in the face of every breath

The abbreviation COPD, which stands for Chronic Obstructive Pulmonary Disease, conceals a silent war going on inside our lungs. It's more than just chronic coughing and dyspnea; it's an ongoing battle for breathing, a shadow cast by noxious particles and gasses gradually breathed in. It's a tale spun from two threads: the harsh realities of our surroundings and the unseen influence of genetics, which combine to impact millions of lives globally.

Chronic obstructive pulmonary disease (COPD) is a multifactorial illness composed of emphysema and chronic bronchitis. This complex combination creates a unique respiratory picture, characterized by a range of symptoms such as a chronic cough, wheezing sounds in the chest, an abundance of mucus, and the omnipresent problem of dyspnea. Everybody's experience is different, like a brushstroke adding its own hue to the overall picture of COPD.

The Global Initiative for Chronic Obstructive Lung Disease (GOLD) intervenes in recognition of this diversity, acting as a beacon of hope amidst the mist. Their evidence-based guidelines serve as a source of unity for the medical community, bringing them together in the pursuit of diagnosing, treating, and ultimately preventing COPD. We can negotiate this difficult terrain with their help, enabling patients and medical professionals to battle for survival together.

Consider breathing as an inward struggle rather than a simple act. For patients who have COPD, this is the reality, once-healthy lungs become enmeshed in inflammation, causing their airways to contract like small fists. People pant for air and feel as though their breath has been stolen as a result of this cascading effect that cripples the vital dance between carbon dioxide and oxygen. Even the most basic activities become enormous undertakings as COPD tightens its hold, endangering everyday living and independence in the process.

COPD is a lung condition that affects millions of people worldwide, including more than 16 million Americans. Because of the narrowing and inflammation of the lungs' airways, breathing becomes difficult. Even simple activities like walking might become challenging. Unbelievably, despite the fact that many Americans are unaware they have COPD, it is the third most common cause of death in the country.

The key to maintaining good lung health and preventing COPD is understanding what can harm your lungs. As the primary offender, giving up smoking is the best course of action. Chemicals, dust, and fumes from the job or house might also harm your lungs. Even though some people are genetically predisposed to COPD, they can still take precautions to maintain their health. It's also critical to stay away from anything that irritates your lungs, such as air pollution and secondhand smoke.

It seems as though a person with COPD needs assistance to maintain their lungs functioning properly. This is where many therapies, such as a toolkit for breathing, are useful. Bronchodilators work by relaxing the muscles in the airways, creating microscopic openings that allow air to pass through more freely.They are inhalers, which are similar to lung-freshening puffs. At times, there may be mild inflammation of the lungs, which impedes breathing.Steroids inhaled have the calming, breathing-issue-easing effects of firemen.

Sometimes bronchodilators and steroids are mixed into a single convenient inhaler, providing a double dose of support for maintaining open airways and reducing inflammation. There may not be enough oxygen in the blood when COPD worsens.This is where oxygen treatment helps, giving your body a direct source of oxygen to support optimal performance.

Breathing becomes difficult for a person with COPD during a flare-up, which is similar to an unexpected storm striking their lungs. Exacerbations, or "flare-ups," require immediate medical intervention. They are frequently brought on by illnesses or inhaling dust or fumes. Fortunately, doctors can quiet the storm with medications like these if they receive assistance quickly.

Oral steroids: These medications lessen lung inflammation, just like fire fighters do when they put out a fire.

Antibiotics: These medications go after the nasty guys producing problems if an infection is the cause.

Bronchodilators: Think of these as opening up the airways, making breathing easier like clearing a blocked path

Catching COPD early can be a game-changer. When doctors spot it quickly, you can make lifestyle tweaks that make a big difference, like kicking the smoking habit to the curb. These changes can even add precious years to your life. And because COPD weakens your defenses, regular vaccinations become your secret weapons. Think of them as shields against nasty bugs like the flu and pneumonia, keeping you healthier and happier in the long run.

Bronchodilators: Imagine them as clearing a clogged route to widen the airways and facilitate breathing. Early detection of COPD can have a profound impact. When medical professionals identify it early on, you can make significant lifestyle changes, such as quitting smoking. Even valuable years may be added to your life by these adjustments. Additionally, regular immunisations become your hidden weapons because COPD decreases your defenses. Consider them as long-term protective barriers against infections like the flu and pneumonia, which will ultimately keep you happier and healthier.

It takes more than just medication and medical visits to manage COPD. Maintaining a positive attitude and sound mental health are equally crucial! Amazing tools like online communities, support groups, and even the American Lung Association can help with that. They provide consolation, counsel, and an opportunity to interact with people who are exactly aware of what you're going through; they're like a helping hand. Recall that having positive mental health also affects your physical health!

When it comes to managing COPD, information truly is power. The more knowledge we have about the illness, the more resilience and hope we can instill in ourselves. Together, with healthcare professionals, we can approach the issues one step at a time. Recall that each breath and every attempt constitute a triumph. Together, with hope and cooperation, let's embrace this adventure and navigate the highs and lows of COPD. After all, despite obstacles in the path, life is meant to be lived.

CHAPTER ONE

COPD Awareness

Envision inhaling, but not quite obtaining the necessary amount of air. For those who suffer from COPD, or chronic obstructive pulmonary disease, that is how life can sometimes be. Breathing becomes challenging due to this chronic lung disease, which is similar to having an obstruction in your airway rather than an open one.

Imagine that your lungs are little balloons that expand with each breath. Breath returns easily from healthy lungs. However, the damage and narrowing of the airways caused by COPD makes it more difficult for air to enter and exit the body. This is analogous to balloons becoming smaller and more rigid, making it more difficult to release the air.

COPD Types

COPD comes in two primary forms, Emphysema and Chronic Bronchitis.

Prolonged Bronchitis: Picture yourself with a bothersome houseguest who never goes and who always messes with your air conditioning. That is similar to the effects of chronic bronchitis on the lungs. Your bronchial tubes, which are vital airways that allow air to enter and exit your body, become occupied by inflammation rather than a visitor.

The tubes become inflamed and bloated as a result of this irritation, giving you the sniffles you always have.

Still, that's not all! Plus, this unwanted visitor is bearing a present of extra mucus. Imagine it as if there were slippery slime obstructing your air vents, preventing air from flowing smoothly. What occurs, then, if your airways are obstructed and inflamed at the same time? It should come as no surprise when breathing becomes difficult. You could possibly encounter:

A chronic cough: As if your body is attempting to eject the mucus gathering from your lungs.There are occasions when this cough also produces phlegm.

Breathing difficulties: Picture inhaling through a straw rather than a wide-open pipe.Narrowed airways can feel like that, especially when you're exercising and need more breath.

Your airway's unwanted guest may cause these symptoms, which can make routine tasks feel like climbing a mountain. Fortunately, there are techniques to help control this illness and improve breathing.

Physicians can assist by:

- Reducing the inflammation which is similar to soothing an irate visitor so they won't tamper with your air conditioner.

- Assisting you in eliminating surplus mucus: Imagine it as unclogging the vents to restore unobstructed airflow.

- Suggestions for altering one's lifestyle include staying away from dusty areas and giving up smoking—the biggest party bomber for the lungs.

Remember that with the appropriate treatment, chronic bronchitis is treatable. See your physician, and try not to allow that bothersome visitor dominate your breath.

Emphysema:

With each breath, picture your lungs as millions of tiny balloons that assist you in releasing carbon dioxide and absorbing oxygen. These balloons, known as alveoli, suffer damage and lose their elasticity in emphysema. Breathlessness results from your lungs having a tougher time functioning as a result of this.

What harms this? The primary cause is smoking, although other factors include dust, air pollution, and even heredity.

What is the sensation? As the harm worsens, you may observe:

Breathlessness: This is the most typical symptom, particularly when exercising.

Whistling when breathing is known as wheezing.

Tightness in the chest: As if a band were pressing on your chest.

Fatigue: Lack of oxygen in your body makes you easily tired.

Is a treatment available? Sadly, the answer is no. However, there are methods to control it:

The most crucial step is to ***give up smoking!***

Medication: Breathing can be facilitated by using an inhaler to open your airways.

Breathing techniques and exercises as part of pulmonary rehabilitation.

Oxygen treatment: More oxygen may be helpful in extreme situations.

Lead a healthy lifestyle by avoiding pollutants, dust, and illnesses.

Although emphysema is a chronic condition, it can be managed and a fulfilling life can be had with the correct care and lifestyle modifications. Discuss the best course of action with your physician.

Examining the Pathophysiology of COPD to Reveal Its Inner Workings

Consider the network of airways that comprise your lungs. Cigarette smoke and other irritants function as obstacles in Chronic Obstructive Pulmonary Disease (COPD), producing inflammation and damage that makes breathing difficult. Let's examine how this occurs:

1. **The Attack Starts**: When you inhale toxic irritants, your airways get inflamed. This inflammation is similar to having irate demonstrators obstructing your lungs' main thoroughfares.

2. **Cells Take Up Arms**: In an attempt to rid itself of the irritants, your body releases immune cells, but in

the process, this "fight" actually deteriorates the delicate lining of your airways, much like clefts in a road.

3. Walls Collapse: Your lungs' air sacs, which are in charge of gas exchange, become less flexible and strong, much like deteriorating bridges giving way. This restricts the free passage of air.

4. Mucus Mess: Inflammation also leads to increased mucus production in the airways, which resembles a dense fog obstructing the roads. Breathing becomes more difficult due to this mucous on top of the damaged roads.

Symptoms: All of this harm results in the typical COPD symptoms, which include:

Recurrent cough: Your body is attempting to get rid of the mucous accumulation.

More mucus: Thicker phlegm may be observed.

Breathlessness: The sensation of not obtaining enough air, akin to everything moving slowly due to traffic congestion.

Breathing problems: Even simple tasks become challenging.

Retaliating: Despite the fact that COPD cannot be cured, it can still be managed by;

Stopping the attacks: Giving up smoking is essential!It is comparable to removing obstacles.

Inflammation reduction: Drugs can assist in lowering the "protest" in your respiratory tract.

Building the roads again: Pulmonary rehabilitation activities help to strengthen and enhance breathing.

Modifications to lifestyle: Remaining healthy and avoiding irritants is similar to maintaining a well-kept highway system.

Knowing about COPD enables us to respond. Knowing the procedures, we can collaborate with medical professionals to treat the ailment and enhance the lives of those impacted.

Knowing Who, What, and Why COPD Is There:

A chronic cough alone is not the only symptom of chronic obstructive pulmonary disease (COPD). It's a major global health issue that affects millions of people, especially those over 40. Even while smoking is frequently portrayed as the bad guy, the narrative doesn't end there. The causes of COPD are varied, and its effects extend well beyond a smoker's habit.

Think of your lungs as a huge network of highways, with every breath representing an exchange of oxygen. This network is disrupted by several obstacles in COPD, causing it to deteriorate. Let's investigate who is causing these obstructions:

Workplace Dangers: In addition to smoking, other factors that can contribute to COPD include breathing in dust, fumes, and chemicals. Farmers, miners, and construction workers are particularly exposed to dangers all the time.

The Hold of Air Pollution: Our air isn't always pure. Long-term exposure to contaminated air, particularly in cities, creates additional barriers that obstruct the free passage of oxygen.

Genes: A genetic predisposition to COPD makes some people more prone to developing the ailment, similar to a curve in the road.

The Divergent Paths: There are two primary kinds of COPD, and each has unique difficulties.

Prolonged Bronchitis: Imagine your motorways restricted because of ongoing inflammation. Coughing and congestion result from mucus buildup, which is like construction slowing down traffic.

Emphysema: This is where the road's structure itself deteriorates. Air sacs become less elastic, like crumbling bridges that impede airflow and make breathing difficult.

The Ripple Effect: COPD affects much more than just breathing problems. It impacts everyday tasks, slumber, and even psychological health. It affects every part of your journey and is comparable to the obstacles that cause traffic delays throughout your entire life.

The Path to Hope: Despite the absence of a treatment, hope remains. We can respond by comprehending the complexities:

Changes in Lifestyle: Giving up smoking should be the first focus, as it is the major obstacle to overcome. Your lungs stay robust and resilient when you exercise and maintain a good diet.

Medical Interventions: Drugs can help open airways and reduce inflammation, such as by facilitating the smooth operation of traffic lights.

Ongoing Support: People with COPD may take charge of their condition and confidently traverse their path with the help of education, pulmonary rehabilitation, and support groups.

Although living with COPD is a complicated path, we can help people live more full lives and breathe easier by helping them recognise the obstacles and services that are out there. We can travel this path together, removing each obstacle as we go.

CHAPTER TWO

Identifying COPD

The process of diagnosing Chronic Obstructive Pulmonary Disease (COPD) is laborious and includes a thorough assessment of medical history, risk factors, and multiple diagnostic procedures. This investigation explores the essential components of diagnosing COPD, such as imaging methods, spirometry, pulmonary function tests, arterial blood gas (ABG) analysis, and health history evaluation.

Risk factors and medical history

A comprehensive review of one's medical history is the first step towards a COPD diagnosis. Information regarding the patient's symptoms, way of life, and exposure to risk factors is gathered by medical specialists. Important components include a history of smoking, a persistent cough, dyspnea, occupational exposure to pollutants, and a family history of respiratory disorders. Knowing the patient's past helps with focused diagnostic efforts and offers insightful information about possible triggers.

Studies on Pulmonary Function

Studies on pulmonary function are essential for assessing lung function and making the diagnosis of COPD. The main test for determining how much and how quickly air is breathed in or out is spirometry. Spirometry measures lung capacity, airflow restriction, and other vital characteristics by forcing the patient to exhale into a device known as a spirometer. The diagnosis of COPD is aided by reduced airflow and poor lung function seen in spirometry findings.

Spirometry and Analysis of ABG

Arteriovenous blood gas (ABG) analysis, which evaluates blood oxygen and carbon dioxide levels, is a useful adjunct to spirometry. The effectiveness of gas exchange in the lungs can be understood from the ABG values. ABG measurement frequently shows elevated carbon dioxide and decreased oxygen levels in COPD patients, indicating poor respiratory function. This combined method improves the precision of the diagnosis and indicates the seriousness of the ailment.

Imaging as well as Screening

Imaging investigations are essential for the diagnosis of COPD because they make lung structures visible and help spot any abnormalities. X-rays of the chest are frequently used to evaluate the presence of infections, lung illnesses, or structural abnormalities. More comprehensive images are provided by high-resolution computed tomography (HRCT) scans, which help distinguish between emphysema and chronic bronchitis and provide a closer look at lung structures.

Diagnostic evaluations benefit from screening instruments like the modified Medical Research Council (mMRC) dyspnea scale and the COPD Assessment Test (CAT). By measuring how COPD affects a patient's day-to-day activities, these tools assist clinicians in determining the total disease burden and developing treatment strategies that take it into account.

A complex process is used to diagnose COPD, taking into account a patient's medical history, risk factors, and a variety of other tests.

Spirometry and ABG analysis are two pulmonary function investigations that provide quantitative information on lung function and gas exchange, and they are the mainstay of diagnostic efforts. Imaging tests, such HRCT scans and chest X-rays, provide visual information about the structures of the lungs, which can help confirm the diagnosis and assess the degree of lung damage.

Comprehending the COPD diagnostic process highlights the significance of adopting a comprehensive approach that takes into account both objective and clinical data. This thorough assessment guarantees a precise diagnosis, guides treatment choices, and creates a framework for continuing care and assistance for people with COPD.

CHAPTER THREE

Life With COPD

Dyspnea, Prolonged Cough, and Other Issues

People who have Chronic Obstructive Pulmonary Disease (COPD) deal with a variety of difficult symptoms that greatly affect their day-to-day activities. This investigation explores some of the most common symptoms, such as the main complaint of a chronic cough, excessive sputum production, progressive dyspnea, weight loss, and the characteristic barrel chest of emphysema.

The main symptom is a persistent cough

One of the main indicators of COPD is frequently a chronic, ongoing cough. The majority of the time, this cough produces mucus or spit. The respiratory system tries to rid the airways of allergens and extra mucus by producing a cough. The persistent nature of this cough can be physically and psychologically exhausting for those who have COPD, which can have an impact on everyday activities and quality of life.

Excessive sputum production

A hallmark of COPD is excessive sputum production, which exacerbates respiratory symptoms and contributes to a persistent cough. Breathing becomes much harder when there is more mucus in the airways, which can cause further obstruction of the airways. Increasing airway clearance with medication and therapy techniques is a common component of managing sputum production in patients with COPD.

Dyspnea Progressive: Strenuous to Rest:

One progressive and characteristic symptom of COPD is dyspnea, or shortness of breath. People eventually find that even ordinary tasks become difficult, although they are initially felt during physical activity. Breathlessness can occur when doing simple tasks, traveling short distances, or climbing stairs. Dyspnea may worsen during sleep as COPD progresses, which can significantly limit a person's capacity to do daily tasks.

The Consequences of Losing Weight

The increased energy expenditure connected to respiratory difficulties is typically the cause of unintentional weight loss, a common aspect of COPD. Weight reduction is influenced by the respiratory muscles' caloric expenditure and the effort needed to breathe. An additional effect on metabolism may come from the systemic inflammation linked to COPD. Since weight loss can worsen fatigue, weakness, and general health decline, it is a worrisome component of COPD that needs to be addressed.

Emphysema Barrel Chest

A barrel chest develops as a result of structural alterations in the lungs that characterize emphysema, one of the main types of COPD. This happens because the lung tissue no longer has its elastic rebound, which keeps the chest from contracting. The chest looks barrel-shaped because of its larger anteroposterior diameter. The emphysema patient's barrel chest is a visible representation of the anatomical changes in their lungs and can be used as a diagnostic marker.

Dealing with a range of symptoms that significantly affect everyday living is part of having COPD. The complications people encounter are highlighted by symptoms such as weight loss, worsening dyspnea, hyperproduction of sputum, chronic cough, and the characteristic barrel chest of emphysema. To treat these symptoms and improve the general quality of life for individuals managing COPD, effective management measures are essential. These strategies include medications, pulmonary rehabilitation, and lifestyle modifications.

CHAPTER FOUR

Preventive Actions

Maintaining Order and Regularity Disciplined and persistent work is necessary to stop Chronic Obstructive Pulmonary Disease (COPD) from developing and worsening. This investigation explores crucial preventive strategies, highlighting the significance of quitting smoking, avoiding environmental and occupational dangers, the impact of genetic variables, and the cultivation of discipline for long-term lung independence.

Quitting Smoking: An Important Intervention Quitting smoking is the single most important COPD preventative intervention. The main cause of COPD is cigarette smoke, and giving up can greatly reduce the disease's progression. Given the increased risk associated with smoking and secondhand smoke exposure, quitting is an essential step. Support groups, nicotine replacement treatments, and smoking cessation programmes are excellent resources for people starting.

Preventing Environmental and Occupational Hazards

The onset and aggravation of COPD may be linked to environmental risks and occupational exposure to dangerous substances. It is essential to reduce exposure to chemicals, dust, and fumes at work. Using ventilation systems and using masks are two appropriate preventative methods that can drastically lower the incidence of respiratory issues. Preventive actions are also supported by being aware of environmental hazards, such as air quality, and by limiting exposure.

COPD and Genetic Factors

Although smoking is the main cause of COPD, susceptibility to the disease is also influenced by hereditary factors. People who have a family history of respiratory disorders may be more likely to acquire COPD. Individuals can make knowledgeable decisions regarding early intervention and preventive actions by using genetic testing and counseling, which can offer insightful information. Being aware of one's hereditary risk enables people to take preventative measures for their respiratory health.

Handling Chronic Pulmonary Freedom with Discipline

An essential part of successful COPD prevention strategies is discipline. Sustaining a healthy lifestyle with frequent exercise, a balanced diet, and enough hydration is beneficial to respiratory health overall. Complying with prescription drug regimens, visiting the doctor on a regular basis, and treating underlying medical issues early on are all examples of discipline. It is possible to achieve chronic pulmonary freedom and lead a full life free from the limitations of COPD by establishing discipline in daily routines.

COPD prevention strategies necessitate a methodical and uniform approach. Giving up smoking is one of the most important interventions that can change the course of the disease. Preventing or managing the advancement of COPD can be achieved through avoiding occupational and environmental dangers, identifying hereditary variables, and fostering discipline in lifestyle choices.

The dissemination of knowledge and the promotion of proactive measures highlight the significance of discipline in maintaining chronic pulmonary freedom and pave the way for a future in which preventative efforts reduce the burden of COPD.

CHAPTER FIVE

Surviving COPD

Pharmacologic Therapy: Managing Chronic Obstructive Pulmonary Disease (COPD) effectively often entails a combination of pharmacologic therapies customized to each patient's needs. This exploration explores important facets of pharmacologic management, such as the use of bronchodilators, the function of corticosteroids, additional COPD medications, and the particular strategy for managing medication during exacerbations.

Bronchodilators: Short and Long-Acting: Among the most important pharmacologic therapies for COPD management are bronchodilators, which function by relaxing the muscles in the airways to improve airflow. They are divided into two types: short-acting and long-acting bronchodilators. Short-Acting bronchodilators: These offer immediate relief and are frequently used on an as-needed basis to alleviate acute symptoms.

Extended-Duration Bronchodilators: These are recommended for everyday use in order to keep airways open for a prolonged amount of time. Long-acting anticholinergics (LAMAs) and long-acting beta-agonists (LABAs) are two examples. There are also LABA/LAMA combinations available, which give improved efficacy.

The Function of Corticosteroids

Inhaled corticosteroids are an essential part of the management of inflammation associated with COPD. When prescribing them to patients with more severe symptoms, bronchodilators are frequently combined with them. Lung function may be enhanced by inhaled corticosteroids (ICS), which aid in lowering airway inflammation.

Additional COPD medications:
Other drugs are used in addition to bronchodilators and corticosteroids to treat particular characteristics of COPD:

Phosphodiesterase-4 (PDE4) Inhibitors: These drugs, which target airway inflammation, include roflumilast and may be used for some patients with severe COPD.

Mucolytics: Drugs such as guaifenesin thin mucus, facilitating its removal from the respiratory system.

Antibiotics: Antibiotics may be used to treat respiratory infections in cases of exacerbations linked to bacterial infections.

Oxygen Therapy: Supplemental oxygen therapy is essential to maintaining adequate blood oxygen levels in patients with advanced COPD.

Medication Management of Exacerbations:

Handling Medication During Severe Episodes: Managing medicine becomes especially crucial during exacerbations, which are periods when COPD symptoms rapidly intensify. In order to manage increasing inflammation, oral corticosteroids and short-acting bronchodilators are administered more frequently. In the event that a respiratory infection is suspected of being the cause of the exacerbation, antibiotics could be given.

To sum up, pharmacologic therapy is essential for managing COPD since it tries to enhance lung function generally, lessen inflammation, and ease symptoms. A thorough approach is ensured by the customized use of bronchodilators, the addition of corticosteroids, and the evaluation of other drugs. Furthermore, being aware of the particular drugs needed during exacerbations improves one's capacity to preventatively handle acute episodes, which benefits COPD patients generally.

Essential Strategies for Managing COPD Symptoms and Promoting Overall Well-being:

Medication Adherence: As instructed by your healthcare professional, take prescription drugs consistently to manage symptoms and avoid exacerbations. Maintaining a regular medication schedule is essential for controlling COPD symptoms and averting flare-ups. It may seem easy, but it's a useful step that can significantly improve your day-to-day experience.

Consider the drugs you take as instruments to maintain the balance of your respiratory system. To maintain the best potential functioning of your lungs, you need to take your prescriptions, just as a carpenter requires the proper tools to make something.

Establish a Schedule: Establishing a schedule is very vital, everyday, take your prescriptions at the same time. You may associate it with a regular task, such as eating or brushing your teeth. This regimen facilitates the development of a medication-taking habit.

Use aids like pill organizers or smartphone reminders if you ever have trouble remembering things. These can be quite helpful in helping you stay on course. Recall that the stability that these medications offer might be compromised by missing doses or changing your prescription schedule. It's similar to attempting to construct a stable building with missing bricks.

Consistency is key: Maintaining consistency is essential. Talk with your healthcare practitioner if you have any questions regarding the efficacy or adverse effects of your medicine. They are available to assist you in locating the ideal option for your requirements.

You are essentially actively managing your COPD and moving towards a more stable and manageable daily life by adhering to your doctor's recommended drug schedule.

Lifestyle Modifications: Quit smoking if you smoke, and avoid exposure to secondhand smoke. One of the biggest things you can do for your COPD and general health is to stop smoking. It's similar to shutting off a significant respiratory supply.

The practical aspect of it is this: consider smoking to be a bad friend you have been hanging out with. Although it may be difficult to let go, you will benefit from it. If you smoke, think about getting help to stop. To assist you with the process, there are hotlines, counseling services, and even applications available. Recall that you are not traveling alone.

Now, avoiding secondhand smoke is similar to avoiding the toxic friend of someone else. If you are unable to give up smoking immediately, at least make an effort to avoid areas where people are smoking. It's similar to selecting cleaner air to give your lungs a break.

When it comes to doable actions, recognise your triggers. Why do you feel the need to smoke? Knowing this can assist you in substituting other activities for smoking. Gum chewing, a quick stroll, or picking up a hobby are some possible ways to keep your hands and mind busy.

Make your house a smoke-free environment. It's similar to building your lungs a secure sanctuary. Toss out ashtrays, extinguish smoke odors, and open doors to allow in fresh air. If you're worried about gaining weight while quitting, concentrate on eating well and exercising. It's about modifying your lifestyle for the better in order to support your desire to stop.

Recall that stopping is a process, and obstacles may arise. Don't be too hard on yourself if you make a mistake. Take what you can from it and keep on. The longer you abstain from smoking, the better your lungs will be able to recover and manage COPD. For your own wellbeing, it's a journey well worth taking.

Maintain a healthy weight through proper diet and exercise: Feeling your best and treating COPD depend greatly on maintaining a healthy weight. Think of it like maintaining the proper fuel supply and efficient operation of your body's engine.

Take care of your diet first. Consider food as the source of energy for your body. Make sure you consume a healthy variety of nutritious grains, fruits, veggies, and lean meats. It is analogous to adding the proper ingredients to a recipe. See your healthcare practitioner or a nutritionist for specific guidance if you're not sure where to begin.

Controlling portion size is essential: Consider the parts of a puzzle that your meals must fit together perfectly. Your body may be able to manage smaller, more frequent meals. It's similar to distributing your digestive system's burden over the course of the day.

Being hydrated is important: Drinking enough water is just as vital. Keep your body working properly by drinking enough water. Giving your engine the fluids it requires to run smoothly is analogous to doing this.

Exercise: This brings us to the topic of exercise. Finding activities that fit your talents is more important than training for a marathon. All you have to do is do simple exercises like yoga or tai chi, go on short walks, or do light stretches. Consider it like a routine check-up for your body.

See your doctor if you have any questions about what kind of exercise is appropriate for you. They could offer you advice on a good workout regimen. Seeking expert guidance is advisable, much as you wouldn't start a new car without first consulting the owner's manual.

Think about including things you like to do. It's similar to adding enjoyment to your workout regimen, increasing the likelihood that you'll continue. Retaining a healthy weight doesn't need rigorous exercise regimens or rigid diets. It involves changing your lifestyle in a sustainable way to promote your general wellbeing. You can enhance your quality of life and help your body adapt to COPD by providing it with the proper treatment.

Respiratory Rehabilitation: Participating in pulmonary rehabilitation programmes is similar to giving your body a customized workout and improving your general health. It's similar to enrolling in a fitness class, but with a focus on improving lung function and overall health. Consider it a collaborative endeavor with medical professionals serving as your guides.

These programmes typically involve support, instruction, and physical activity. Your respiratory muscles will progressively become stronger as a result of the exercises, which will facilitate better breathing. It's similar to giving your lungs' coordinating muscles focused workout.

The instructional part is similar to learning insider information about how your lungs work and how to take better care of your health. You may pick up energy-saving methods, breathing exercises, and coping mechanisms for common COPD difficulties. Think of it as a comprehensive strategy that addresses your general health as well as your lungs. It's similar to looking after your entire body and mind.

Let's now discuss the useful aspect. Because these programmes are typically overseen, you may be sure that the activities are safe and appropriate for your skill level. It's similar to having a coach who is aware of your unique requirements,maintaining consistency is essential. Don't hesitate to voice your concerns or ask questions to the medical staff during your frequent attendance at the sessions. This is a partnership, and your active participation makes a difference.

Apply the knowledge you gain to your day-to-day activities. You can practice the activities you perform in these programmes at home. It's similar to incorporating an easy-to-follow exercise regimen into your daily schedule.
Recall that the goal of pulmonary rehabilitation is to improve your total quality of life, not just your lung function. You're investing in your health and equipping yourself with the skills you need to effectively manage your COPD by actively engaging in these programmes.

Breathing Techniques: Learning how to breathe correctly is like discovering a hidden weapon that will enable you to control your breathing and breathe more easily. It's important to breathe in a way that supports your lungs and lessens strain, not just to breathe.

First of all, think of it as being similar to learning to play an instrument. Breathing is a skill that may be significantly improved with practice. Simple breathing techniques like slowly inhaling through your nose and exhaling through pursed lips are a good place to start. It is similar to teaching your lungs to breathe in more air and exhale more effectively.

Practice often: Consider it a form of exercise for your breathing muscles. As with any workout regimen, the secret is to be consistent. Every day, dedicate a short period of time to concentrate on your breathing techniques. It's similar to strengthening a particular muscle group,in this case, your lungs,through consistent practice.

These methods then become your go-to resources when you're having trouble breathing. It's similar to carrying a portable cure. Try diaphragmatic breathing, for instance, which involves deep breathing while permitting your diaphragm to fully contract. It functions somewhat like increasing your lung capacity.

Include these strategies in your everyday routine. It resembles forming a brand-new habitual habit. You can engage in mindful breathing while walking, standing, or sitting. It becomes a natural aspect of your breathing and not just an activity.

Never be afraid to seek advice. A respiratory therapist or your healthcare physician can offer specific guidance. It's similar to working with a coach to perfect your technique. Once you have the hang of it, breathing correctly can be a useful tool in your toolbox for managing COPD. By devoting time and energy to these practices, you're giving yourself the tools you need to overcome obstacles and breathe easier.

Nutrition: Eat a healthy, well-balanced diet to maintain your general well-being and vitality. Eating a healthy, well-balanced diet is like feeding your body the right things to keep everything functioning properly, especially if you have COPD. Making decisions that are realistic and improve your general health and energy levels is more important than adhering to rigid restrictions.

Consider your meals as a collaborative effort to enhance your overall health. A wide range of foods, such as fruits, vegetables, entire grains, and lean proteins, should be included. It's like arranging a rainbow of colors on your plate to make sure you get all the important nutrients.

Think about serving sizes: Consider your plate as a pie chart, with distinct areas representing the various food groups. It's important to strike the correct balance, neither too high nor too low. It's similar to adjusting your diet to fulfill your body's requirements without going overboard.
Remain hydrated. It's similar to giving your body the fluids it requires to operate properly to drink enough water. It's a straightforward but crucial component of preserving health and vitality.

See your doctor or a nutritionist if you're unclear about what foods to choose. They can help you make sensible and doable food decisions. It's similar to having a food plan that is customized for your unique health requirements, consider it a lifestyle rather than a diet. Include foods you enjoy, and if you splurge once in a while, don't be too hard on yourself. It's about figuring out a healthy eating pattern that you can stick to.

Think about making easy changes. For instance, choose lean protein sources or whole grains rather than refined grains. It functions similarly to upgrading your fuel to a higher grade for enhanced efficiency. Eating a well-balanced and nutrient-rich diet gives your body the building blocks it needs to manage COPD and stay as energetic as possible, in addition to giving nourishment. It's an important and useful step towards general wellbeing.

Stay Hydrated: Water consumption should be sufficient to support mucus formation and facilitate breathing. In addition to providing your body with the necessary fluids to keep a balanced environment, drinking adequate water is essential for controlling mucus production and facilitating easier breathing in those with COPD.

Imagine that water is the lubrication of a well-oiled machine, which is your body. It's like making sure everything functions properly, including the formation and removal of mucus from your respiratory system, when you maintain an appropriate level of hydration.

Mucus functions as your body's natural defense system, assisting in the removal of allergens from your airways. This mucus is more fluid and easier to remove when you're properly hydrated. It resembles your lungs' internal self-cleaning mechanism. When you make drinking water a habit, practicality enters the picture. Keep a water bottle with you at all times, and sip from it frequently. It's similar to giving your body the continuous supply of fluids it requires to perform at its best.

Make it your daily objective. Set a goal for the amount of glasses or liters you want to drink, but don't worry about exceeding it. It's similar to flowing gently as opposed to going overboard. If you don't think plain water tastes good, try adding some fruit or herb pieces to it. It's similar to enhancing flavor without sacrificing the moisturizing properties. Herbal broths and teas can add to your daily fluid consumption.

Observe the cues your body is sending you. When you experience thirst, it's time to replenish your fluids. It's similar to paying attention to your body's signals and meeting its requirements. Recall that staying hydrated is an easy yet effective way to manage the symptoms of COPD. Drinking enough water is something you can do consciously to benefit your respiratory system, health and facilitate the efficient functioning of your lungs. It's an easy and useful step towards improved breathing and general health.

Manage Stress: Reduce your stress by engaging in stress-reduction practices like yoga, deep breathing, or meditation to lessen the effect of stress on COPD symptoms. Adding stress-reduction strategies to your daily routine can make a huge difference in how well you manage the symptoms of COPD. It's similar to building a tranquil haven for your body and mind, and it can have a big influence on your general wellbeing.

Consider stress as an additional burden your body must bear. It's as if you're releasing that needless load when you engage in practices like yoga, deep breathing, or meditation. These techniques assist in lowering tension, calming your nervous system, and restoring equilibrium. The key to being practical is figuring out what suits you. It's not about spending hours in meditation or learning difficult poses. Begin modestly.

Every day, set aside some time to sit still and concentrate on your breathing. It's similar to taking a little mental vacation from the stress of everyday life. Think about adding these routines to your stress-reduction regimen. For instance, take a few deep breaths if you're feeling overwhelmed. It's similar to pausing and giving your body and mind a break.

Examine some gentle yoga poses or guided meditation techniques; a lot of these may be found online. It is like having a private coach in the convenience of your own home. Find what feels doable and resonates with you.
Maintaining consistency is essential. Similar to strengthening a muscle, it gets more efficient with repetition. Over time, even a short daily commitment can have a significant impact.

Tell your healthcare practitioner about your experience. They can ensure that these methods support and enhance your COPD management plan by providing advice and assistance. It's similar to having an encouraging partner on your path to wellbeing. You're not just addressing the psychological and emotional aspects of COPD by incorporating stress-reduction tactics into your daily life; you're also laying the groundwork for improved general health. It's a doable and empowering step towards stress management and improving your life.

Regular Check-ups: See your doctor for routine checkups to have your condition assessed, treatment programmes modified, and any concerns addressed. Visiting your doctor on a regular basis is like having a road map for controlling your COPD. Consider these visits as milestones that assist in maintaining your health, much as you would schedule routine maintenance on your vehicle to avoid problems later on.

These trips are centered on practicality. Plan them on a regular basis, and even if you feel well, don't skip them. Similar to preventative treatment, it involves identifying possible problems early on and implementing changes before they have a big impact. Your healthcare professional keeps an eye on several elements of your condition during these check-ups. In addition to discussing any changes in your symptoms, they may assess how well your current treatment plan is working and examine your lung function. It functions similarly to a customized health report that directs your future actions.

Talk candidly and freely about your experiences. Tell us about any new symptoms or difficulties you've encountered. It's similar to giving your medical staff the information they need to customize your treatment plan to meet your changing needs.

Make inquiries: It resembles a dialogue rather than a one-sided communication. Recognise any necessary lifestyle changes, anticipated side effects, and your treatment strategy. You can now take an active role in managing your COPD thanks to this clarity. If you're prescribed medicine, take it as instructed and talk to your doctor about any worries or difficulties you're having. Finding a schedule that works for your lifestyle may help you be more practical in this regard and make adherence easier.

Think of these examinations as group discussions. Your medical professional is available to assist you. Speak up if something isn't working or if you have questions regarding the course of your treatment. It's similar to adjusting until the melody is just perfect while fine-tuning an instrument.

Regular check-ups allow you to actively control your COPD rather than just keep an eye on it. It's a sensible and crucial step to keeping your health, avoiding issues, and making the most out of your COPD journey.

Avoid Respiratory Irritants: Reduce your exposure to allergies, occupational dangers, and environmental contaminants that might exacerbate the symptoms of COPD. In particular while controlling COPD, lowering your exposure to allergens, occupational dangers, and environmental contaminants is like building a barrier for your lungs. Not shunning the outside world entirely is the goal; rather, sensible decisions should be made to reduce possible triggers.

Begin with your living area. Think of it as your haven. Maintain good ventilation, and if you can, utilize air purifiers to remove toxins from the air. It's similar to setting up a hygienic, ventilated space to maintain your respiratory wellness. Refrain from smoking and inhaling smoke. Giving up smoking is a big step if you smoke. Please ask anyone who is smoking near you to go outside. It's similar to making the decision to inhale cleaner air, which eases the burden on your lungs.

Keep yourself updated about the local air quality. If the pollution level is excessive, you might want to stay indoors or modify your outdoor activities. It's similar to checking the weather forecast and modifying your plans according to the present situation. Recognise and control the allergies in your house. Keeping pets out of bedrooms, choosing hypoallergenic bedding, and doing routine cleaning can all be helpful. It's similar to designing a space that reduces possible respiratory problem triggers.

If your job exposes you to chemicals, dust, or other hazards, talk to your employer about what safety measures you may take. It can involve changing your workspace or donning safety gear. It's similar to taking actionable measures to guarantee a safer workplace. Consider donning a mask while engaging in outdoor activities to help filter out airborne pollutants. It's similar to donning armor to protect oneself from possible irritants when going for walks or other outdoor activities.

Pay attention to your body. Take note of any situations or activities that seem to exacerbate your symptoms and make the necessary adjustments. It's similar to choosing decisions that promote your body's health and acting as its advocate.
Reducing exposure is a proactive and realistic way to manage COPD. You're protecting the health of your lungs and improving your quality of life by making your surroundings aware of any triggers.

Vaccinations: To avoid respiratory infections, make sure you are up to date on your vaccinations, especially the flu and pneumonia shots. Maintaining current vaccines is like wearing a barrier over your respiratory system; this is particularly crucial for COPD patients. It's a sensible method of preventing respiratory infections, which can have significant hazards, rather than just avoiding vaccinations.

Obtain the flu shot first. Think of it as an annual tradition, similar to fastening your seatbelt before you drive. People with COPD are more vulnerable to the flu, and vaccination offers vital protection.

Plan it for the autumn, before the flu season begins. Vaccines against pneumonia provide an additional line of defense. In contrast to the flu shot, you might not require them annually. You will receive guidance on the proper timetable from your healthcare practitioner. Consider it an investment in your respiratory health for the long run.

The important thing is to be practical. Put immunization dates in your calendar or use your phone to create reminders. It's similar to making sure your shield of defense is always current. To help you keep on schedule, certain pharmacies also provide easy vaccination services. When talking about vaccinations, let your healthcare practitioner know that you have COPD. They can modify suggestions in accordance with your particular requirements. It is comparable to getting a customized immunization schedule based on your current state of health.

Remember to receive additional regular vaccines. For example, confirm that your tetanus shot is current. It's like maintaining the all-around quality of your health defenses. Talk to your healthcare practitioner about your reservations if you have any about immunisations. They can offer information to clear up any misunderstandings and support you in making wise choices. It's similar to having a talk to make sure you're comfortable with the decisions you're making with your health.

You can take steps to lower your risk of respiratory infections by making sure you are up to date on your vaccines. It's an easy-to-use, practical measure that makes a big difference in your overall health and helps you manage your COPD efficiently.

Oxygen Therapy: Use extra oxygen as indicated if required to maintain sufficient blood oxygen levels. If prescribed, using supplemental oxygen is like giving your body the extra help it needs to keep the blood's oxygen levels at a healthy level, which is essential for managing COPD. It's a useful instrument that can significantly enhance your daily life rather than a burden.

Think of extra oxygen as a breathing aid that is helpful. If your doctor prescribes it, make sure you carefully follow their directions. It's similar to having a customized plan to make sure you get the appropriate quantity of oxygen for your needs.

Incorporating oxygen utilization into your lifestyle is practical. Make it a habit to wear your oxygen as directed if you require it for activities or sleep. Consider it analogous to donning spectacles to improve vision - oxygen becomes a vital part of your everyday routine.

Recognise the equipment. Discover how to operate and care for your oxygen equipment. It is similar to familiarizing yourself with any tool that simplifies your life. Please do not hesitate to contact the supplier or your healthcare physician with any questions or concerns. Make a plan if you're going anywhere. Mobility may be facilitated by portable oxygen tanks or concentrators. It's similar to having a trustworthy friend who lets you keep your independence and partake in different hobbies.

Open up to people in your vicinity. Tell your friends, family, and coworkers if you're taking extra oxygen. It's a proactive decision for improved health rather than a restriction. Tell them how important it is and how they can help you. Check your oxygen levels frequently. While some gadgets have built-in monitors, others could need a different device. It's similar to making sure your body's oxygen tank is always full by monitoring the gasoline indicator.

Recall that getting extra oxygen helps you live a more active and satisfying life. It's a tool. It's a sensible step to make sure your body gets the oxygen it needs to perform at its best, not a show of weakness. Accept it as a partner on your path to successful COPD management......

CHAPTER SIX

Inhale, Concentrate on Living.

Modifications to Lifestyle

In order to effectively manage Chronic Obstructive Pulmonary Disease (COPD), one must adopt lifestyle changes that put respiratory health first. This investigation explores the topic of breath-focused living and covers topics such as personalized care plans, holistic approaches to COPD management, the importance of exercise and diet, and the critical components of mental and emotional health.

Comprehensive COPD Remedies

The interdependence of the physical, mental, and emotional facets of health is recognised in holistic approaches to COPD. Acupuncture, yoga, and breathing techniques are examples of integrative therapies that can enhance medical treatments. These all-encompassing COPD therapies seek to improve respiratory function, lower stress levels, and increase general well-being.

Strategies for Personalized Care

Personalized care solutions are crucial because each person with COPD manifests differently. Individuals and healthcare providers must work together to customize management regimens to meet personal needs. A key component of providing effective, individualized care is evaluating lifestyle circumstances, comprehending individual triggers, and setting reasonable goals.

Exercise and Diet for People with COPD

A vital part of helping people with COPD is nutrition. Essential nutrients can be obtained via a diet that is well-balanced and abundant in fruits, vegetables, lean meats, and whole grains. Staying properly hydrated is also essential to preserving lung health.

Exercise on a regular basis is essential for managing COPD. Engaging in physical activity enhances endurance and fortifies the respiratory muscles.

Including both strength training activities and cardio exercises, such as cycling or walking, improves overall fitness. Programmes for pulmonary rehabilitation provide regimens of structured exercise customized for persons with COPD.

Emotional and Psychological Health

Addressing the psychological and emotional components of COPD symptoms is just as important as treating the physical ones. People with chronic illnesses frequently experience anxiety and depression, which lowers their quality of life overall. Counseling, mindfulness exercises, and support groups can all help with stress management and emotional wellbeing.

Comprehensive COPD care requires open conversation regarding mental health with medical professionals. For people with COPD, breath-focused living includes holistic approaches, individualized care plans, attention to exercise and diet, and a focus on mental and emotional health. Adopting a holistic perspective on health enables people to face the obstacles posed by COPD with fortitude and self-determination. People can promote a happy and balanced lifestyle by combining medical interventions with lifestyle changes irrespective of the limitations of COPD.

CHAPTER SEVEN

Optimal Health for COPD

Techniques for the Best COPD Wellness

For people with Chronic Obstructive Pulmonary Disease (COPD), optimal wellbeing entails using all-encompassing management strategies that uplift life, deal with day-to-day difficulties, and foster resilience to get beyond setbacks. This investigation explores important tactics for reaching and maintaining the best possible COPD wellbeing.

All-encompassing Management Techniques

A comprehensive and all-encompassing management strategy that includes medical interventions, lifestyle modifications, and mental well-being is necessary for optimal COPD wellbeing. A holistic approach is ensured by working together with healthcare specialists to customize a management plan that is unique to each patient's needs. To improve general respiratory health, this involves pulmonary rehabilitation, integrative therapies, individualized care plans, and medication management.

Taking Charge of Life with COPD

Developing a sense of control and self-efficacy is essential to empowering life with COPD. Empowerment is facilitated by knowledge of the condition, awareness of triggers, and active involvement in the management process. Participating in support networks—whether via support groups or establishing connections with peers going through comparable struggles—offers a priceless feeling of shared experiences and community.

Handling Everyday Difficulties

The everyday struggles posed by COPD might vary from coping with symptoms to overcoming restrictions on physical activity. Creating constructive coping mechanisms entails adjusting to these difficulties while keeping an optimistic outlook. This can entail setting boundaries for oneself, using assistive technology when required, and coming up with creative solutions for chores. Adaptive methods make life easier on a daily basis.

Overcoming Difficulties and Being Resilient

In order to overcome the challenges posed by COPD, resilience is essential. Developing an attitude that values persistence and adaptation is a key component in building resilience. Overcoming challenges involves recognising setbacks, drawing lessons from them, and concentrating on solutions. Resilience is further strengthened by participating in joyful and meaningful activities, which promotes a proactive approach to managing COPD.

The key components of optimal COPD wellbeing are accepting holistic management techniques, empowering living with COPD, creating useful coping mechanisms for day-to-day struggles, and building resilience to go past setbacks. People with COPD can live happy, full lives that put their general well-being first by combining medical advice with self-determination, resilience, and a resilient mindset.

CHAPTER EIGHT

Managing COPD Difficulties

Realistic Perspectives

Managing Chronic Obstructive Pulmonary Disease (COPD) calls for practical knowledge that includes daily living advice, efficient management techniques, and methods to improve overall quality of life. This investigation offers insightful information to those looking to confidently conquer COPD obstacles.

Daily Life Advice

The following helpful hints for managing daily life with COPD can greatly enhance the experience:

Pacing of Activities: To preserve energy, divide work into manageable chunks and provide time for relaxation in between.

Optimizing the Environment: Make sure that living areas are clear of any respiratory irritants and have adequate ventilation. If required, use air purifiers.

Assistive Devices: To promote mobility and independence, think about utilizing assistive devices like walkers or portable oxygen concentrators.

Drink enough water to help thin mucus and facilitate its removal from the airways.

Strategies for managing COPD that work

Putting into practice efficient management techniques is essential for overcoming COPD's challenges:

Medication Adherence: Carefully adhere to the recommended dosage schedules and let your healthcare providers know if you have any questions or concerns about any side effects.

Frequent Exercise: To improve respiratory and general physical health, participate in customized exercise regimens that emphasize both aerobic and strength training activities.

Investigate pulmonary rehabilitation programmes that provide people with COPD with supervised exercise, instruction, and assistance.

Healthy Nutrition: To promote general health and sustain energy levels, adopt a nutrient-rich, well-balanced diet.

Improving Living Quality

The following are some methods to improve the quality of life for people with COPD:

1) Establish social ties with family, friends, and support groups to fend off feelings of loneliness and advance mental health.

2) Mindfulness Practices: To reduce the tension and anxiety brought on by COPD, combine mindfulness with relaxation methods.

3) Adaptive Techniques: To preserve independence, adopt adaptive techniques including making trip plans in advance and utilizing gadgets to make everyday chores easier.

Getting Over Obstacles with Self-Belief

To confidently overcome COPD obstacles, one must:

Education: Keep up with the latest developments in COPD care and treatment options by educating yourself on a regular basis.

Communication: Keep lines of communication open by talking about difficulties and actively engaging in the management plan with healthcare providers.

Positivity: Instead of concentrating on your limits, adopt an optimistic outlook by concentrating on what you can do. Appreciate your little progress along the way.

Useful advice for overcoming the obstacles posed by COPD includes day-to-day living techniques, efficient management approaches, and efforts to improve general quality of life. People with COPD can maximize their everyday experiences and cultivate a positive view on their journey with this chronic condition by confidently putting these thoughts into practice.

CHAPTER NINE

Successfully Managing COPDA

Trip Towards Liveliness

Taking control of your life with chronic Obstructive Pulmonary Disease (COPD) is the first step towards living a vital life. This extensive manual attempts to offer vital information to people who, in spite of the obstacles presented by COPD, are looking for robust health and optimal living.

Managing Chronic Obstructive Pulmonary Disease in Daily Life

Living with COPD requires a proactive, all-encompassing attitude to everyday living.

Knowledge Empowerment: Keep learning about COPD and keep up to date on symptoms, available treatments, and lifestyle modifications.

Self-Management Skills: Acquire the ability to self-monitor, spot early warning indicators of exacerbations, and put effective symptom management techniques into practice.

Collaborative Care: Encourage cooperative ties with medical professionals, taking an active role in the creation and modification of the COPD treatment plan.

An All-Inclusive Manual for Optimal Living

A thorough manual for living as optimally as possible with COPD includes a number of aspects:

Healthcare Team Collaboration: To develop a cohesive and successful strategy for managing COPD, form a solid alliance with medical specialists, such as pulmonologists, respiratory therapists, and support personnel.

Lifestyle Modifications: To promote general well being and improve respiratory health, adopt lifestyle modifications such as proper diet, regular exercise, and stress reduction.

Novel therapy Options: To keep up with developments in COPD care, investigate novel therapy options and developing therapies in cooperation with medical professionals.

Essentials of COPD for Optimal Health

Among the necessities for thriving health in the face of COPD are:

Patient advocacy entails standing up for oneself during the management process, actively participating in healthcare choices, and obtaining second opinions.

Embracing Support Systems: To share experiences, exchange wisdom, and promote emotional well-being, cultivate a network of support that includes friends, family, and other COPD fighters.

Setting and Achieving Goals: To maintain a sense of vitality, set reasonable goals, acknowledge and celebrate accomplishments, and concentrate on enjoyable and fulfilling pursuits.

Living well with chronic COPD requires learning to live with it, learning how to follow a detailed roadmap to optimal living, and realizing what is necessary for vibrant health. It's a path towards vitality. Through the integration of knowledge, self-management techniques, collaborative care, lifestyle modifications, and an optimistic outlook, people with COPD can effectively navigate their journey towards optimal well-being with resilience, vigor, and a positive outlook.

END NOTE

Taking a thoughtful and all-encompassing approach to well-being is necessary to empower your journey with Chronic Obstructive Pulmonary Disease (COPD). Being able to answer basic questions regarding COPD, its symptoms, available treatments, and possible lifestyle modifications is the first step towards being empowered. Your ability to navigate the problems that COPD may offer is strengthened by your proactive understanding of the condition and your continued education about it.

One important aspect of empowerment is taking an active role in your care. This includes learning how to effectively manage symptoms on one's own, identifying early warning indicators of exacerbations, and putting self-management techniques into practice. Your unique needs and preferences will be taken into account when you work closely with your healthcare team, which includes respiratory therapists and pulmonologists, to establish a cohesive and successful approach to managing COPD.

A thorough manual on living as optimally as possible with COPD covers a range of topics. It entails changing behaviors that promote general well-being, including adopting a balanced diet, getting regular exercise that is appropriate for your level of ability, and learning how to effectively manage stress. By keeping up with new developments in COPD care and consulting with your healthcare professionals, you can make sure that your care plan changes as the condition is treated.

In the context of COPD, patient advocacy—actively engaging in healthcare decisions, obtaining second views when necessary, and remaining involved in the management process—is essential for vigorous health. Building a solid support system with friends, family, and other COPD fighters is a great way to exchange insights, exchange stories, and promote emotional health.

Setting and achieving goals becomes essential to living well with COPD. You support a feeling of vitality and purpose by setting attainable objectives, acknowledging accomplishments, and concentrating on pursuits that make you happy and fulfilled. A positive outlook is crucial because your road with COPD is distinct and ever-changing. Remind yourself that you are not alone on this path. You may greatly improve your general well-being by reaching out to support networks and recognising and appreciating your little accomplishments along the route.

A comprehensive and cooperative strategy that includes information mastery, active engagement in care, lifestyle modifications, staying up to date on available treatments, patient advocacy, and cultivating an optimistic outlook is necessary to empower your journey with COPD. Despite the challenges posed by COPD, you can achieve resilience, vigor, and an enhanced quality of life by adopting these aspects.

www.ingramcontent.com/pod-product-compliance
Lightning Source LLC
Chambersburg PA
CBHW070756250726
48662CB00004B/1830